Dr EDWARD LAVAL

The

Illness and Death

of

General Gallieni

Academic Library PERRIN & Co.

Translated and Edited by John Phillips, MD

Dʳ EDOUARD LAVAL

La
Maladie et la mort

DU

Général Gallieni

Prix : 2 fr. 50   *Librairie académique PERRIN et Cⁱᵉ*

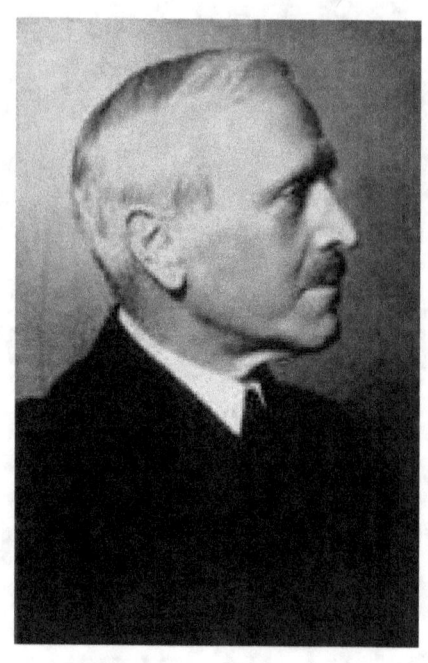

Edouard Laval
1871-1965

Chief of Medicine, St Jean de Dieu, Paris
4th Bureau French HQ American Expeditionary Forces
Distinguished Service Medal, United States Army, 1919
Author, *Memories of a Staff Army Physician*, 1932

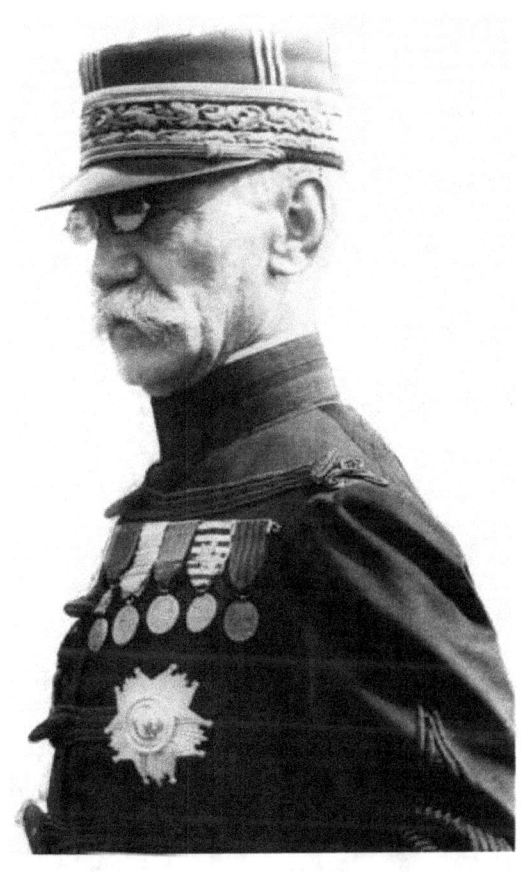

Gen. Joseph Simon Gallieni
1848-1916
1886, Governor, the Sudan
1896, Governor, Madagascar
1905, Commander, 14th Corps, Lyon
Mil. Governor of Paris, 1914
Minister of War, 1915-1916

TABLE OF CONTENTS

Editor's Note

Dr. Edouard Laval was already a published author in military medicine when he became personal physician to General Joseph Gallieni, the so-called 'Savior of Paris', in 1915. Laval was positioned, therefore, to chronicle Gallieni's long struggle with urinary difficulties and eventual demise after prostate surgery in 1916. Gallieni's death shocked all of France. Laval wrote the book, which is part memoir and part homage, in hopes that the facts of the case would dispel the conspiracy theories and rumors surrounding the General's demise and which swirled about Paris for years. The book was published just once, in 1920, by Perrin et Cie, the famed French history and biography press, and sold cheaply in the small, paperback style so common in the little shops and *bouquinistes* that surrounded the Seine. Laval's book can still be found (for just a few more Euros than its original price) but is held by just 6 libraries around the world. The current translation presented here is the work's first in English, reproduced in its original 12 x 19 cm size, and in a large font reminiscent of the original typeface. For comparison, and as an homage to Laval in the style of a *synopsis*, his introductory pages in French are presented opposite their English counterparts. I wish to thank my colleague, Professor Bernard Seguy, MD, AIHP, the famed gynecologic surgeon, the Sage of Nice, for help with some of the subtle delicacies of Laval's writing.   JLP

i

AVANT-PROPOS

———

Dans la chambre où sont écrites ces
lignes flotte la grande ombre du Général
Gallieni. En fermant les yeux je le vois
encore sur le lit où il était couché, à la
place où se trouve ma table, lorsqu'il me
fit appeler, le 17 avril 1914. Il ressentait
alors la première atteinte de l'affection
qui devait peser si lourdement sur la fin
de sa vie. Après l'intervention très simple
usitée en pareille circonstance, les fonc-
tions redevinrent normales et, au bout de
quelques jours, le Général reprit sa vie

PREFACE

In the room where these notes are written, is the great shadow of General Gallieni. Closing my eyes I can still see him on the bed where he lay, the place where my table is now when I was summoned to him on 17 April 1914. At that time he first felt the attack of the disease that must have weighed so heavily on him at the end of his life. After a simple and straight forward intervention, his functions became normal again, and after a few days, the General resumed his usual life by following and observing a few precautions.

habituelle moyennant l'observation de quelques précautions.

En juillet, il quittait son appartement de la rue Dupont-des-Loges, pour se retirer dans sa propriété de la Gabelle près de Saint-Raphaël, où il se préparait à jouir en famille d'un repos légitimement gagné, lorsqu'il fut frappé du deuil le plus cruel : la mort d'une femme qu'il adorait. Quelques heures après, c'était la déclaration de guerre de l'Allemagne. Il regagnait aussitôt la capitale pour se mettre à la disposition du gouvernement. Celui-ci, on le sait, ne tardait pas à le nommer Gouverneur et Commandant en chef des armées de Paris.

Pendant toute la période qui s'est écoulée des derniers jours d'août 1914 au 29 octobre 1915, la maladie qui avait fait

THE DEATH OF GENERAL GALLIENI

In July he was leaving his apartment in the Rue Dupont-des-Loges, to retire to his property in the Gabelle, near Saint-Raphaël, where he was preparing to enjoy a relaxing break with family well deserved, when he was struck by the grief of a most cruel death of the woman whom he adored. A few hours later, came the declaration of war on Germany. He returned as soon as possible to the capital-to make himself available to the government. This, as we know, was when he was soon appointed to be the Governor and Commander-in-Chief of the Army of Paris.

Throughout the period between the last days of August 1914 to the 29th of October, 1915, the illness which he had first developed

sa première apparition en avril 1914 et s'était réveillée se manifesta par des troubles qui exigèrent des soins et un traitement parfois fort énergiques, comme me l'expliqua le Général lui-même, lorsque je le vis dans son cabinet du lycée Duruy au mois de mai 1915, et comme me l'a confirmé le Dr Minet qui veillait alors sur sa santé. Mais c'est surtout pendant son séjour au Ministère que le Général Gallieni vit son affection s'aggraver d'une façon irrésistiblement progressive, au point que l'intervention représentât la seule issue d'une telle situation. Je voudrais précisément essayer de tracer, d'une plume aussi simple et aussi fidèle que possible, l'évolution de cette maladie pendant les derniers mois de la vie du Général. Lorsque le lecteur connaîtra dans

in April 1914, and which was occasionally exacerbated by stress, appeared to demand constant attention and treatments, some of which were very strong, as explained to me by the General himself, when I saw him in his office at the Duruy school in the month of May, 1915, and as confirmed to me by Dr. Minet, who was then attending to his health. But it was during his time in the Ministry, that General Gallieni saw that his condition had unremittingly deteriorated in such a way, that it was now irresistibly clear that some intervention would represent the only way out of his situation. I resolved then to set out and document with a pen, trying to be as simple yet as accurate as possible, the evolution of the disease during the last months of the General's life.

ses détails la longue souffrance physique
et morale que subit alors le Général Gallieni, il verra se dresser plus grande
encore, s'il se peut, la silhouette de
ce grand soldat.

THE DEATH OF GENERAL GALLIENI

When the reader thus knows the details of what physical and mental sufferings General Gallieni long experienced, the silhouette of this great soldier will, if possible, be even greater still.

I

AT THE MINISTRY OF WAR

During my period of leave, General Gallieni received me in the department of the Ministry on December 9, 1915. From the first glance upon entering his vast room where he was alone, I was dismayed at how he had physical changed since I had seen him the previous May: He had lost weight, his skin yellowish; he appeared tired, and this in a sort of man - who had once radiated so strongly, who had been so active — there was now a sort of lassitude, a shade of dejection. Early into our conversation, he explained that his health was bad: the life that was now imposed upon him did not suit him or his expectations.

"I worked", he said, "as one can imagine when the Germans advanced on Paris and through the Battle of the Marne. What I had to do was really hard. I barely ate or slept at all. And also, it was so sad to say: 'That this poor Paris will perhaps fall into the hands of the Germans!' "

This sentence of compassion was so beautiful in its simplicity that it is somewhat reminiscent of that which Joan of Arc was said to have cried, "God will you thus let so die the poor people of Compiegne?"

And he continued:

"I had to use every spare moment to its maximum. I would have had three months off to recharge my batteries and then back to it... Finally, I vowed to just keep walking, so goes the saying, until I drop...

"Jusqu'a bout!"[1] I can still hear him say adding "I will die for the task at hand"... It is the only death I wish..." Then, after a pause: "How well do you think I am doing? Consider that six weeks ago I could walk outside, rain or shine, any time of day... Ah! I did not want to be Minister ... I knew that this job would kill me...Finally, the burden fell upon me, and I accepted and obeyed."

---

[1] *"Up to the very end"*, the defiant pledge that Gallieni gave to all Parisians, to defend the city in the face of imminent encirclement in 1914. The phrase was long associated with Gallieni thereafter and served as a clarion call for French patriotism throughout the War.

The General then said to me, as Dr. Minet had so done for him shortly before the War, that it would be nice for me to attend to his health now, which I done for some time in the past. I appreciated his confidence and assured him of my devotion. Then, to fill me in on the medical nature of his current situation, we agreed that Dr. Minet and I would meet with him the following December 10th at 2100 hours, the only time of day when we knew we would not be disturbed.

At the appointed hour, the General received us in his bedroom, standing, leaning against his bed, biting on his cigarette, his face less tired than yesterday, but still pale and thin.

"Oh my poor Laval," he exclaimed when he saw me, during his last days as Minister of War.

'We talk about the toil imposed on us by the Cabinet meetings, as he once said, during which his colleagues who seemed to be "screwed to their seats", while he himself suffered not being able to get up at all.

"It lasts far too long", he reflected. "What's there to be said? Sadly, very little in reality. Oh, if it were not for the Fatherland! It seems that I

4

give her my service, yet I did not look after myself. I did my time... To me, this is much the same as with my health. I would do anything, until death itself comes, perhaps suddenly, perhaps positioned as a soldier in the trenches..."

"Finally, here," remembering the task at hand. "I'm appointing you to my office," he said, turning to me. But one could see rising from him immediately a bit of the spirit of a man of such high consciousness: he begins to hesitate, because he would hate to commit a physician to deal solely with his person alone. His ordinance officer, Captain Charbonnel, explains then to him that, at the time of his predecessors, Messimy[2], and then Millerand[3], a military doctor was part of the personal staff of the Minister, and that this position currently free, could clearly be assigned to me. As my official job, in the Cabinet, would be to take care of all the affairs of the Health Service, I would be able, at the same time, to attend to the Minister's health.

---

[2] Adolphe Messimy (1869-1935), French Minister of War, 1911-12
[3] Alexandre Millerand (1859-1943), French Minister of War, 1914-1915

It was a compelling argument. "Well, so that's understood, eh?" he concluded. And he added: "Moreover, Laval has been at the front since the beginning of the war, and it is just as appropriate to come here."

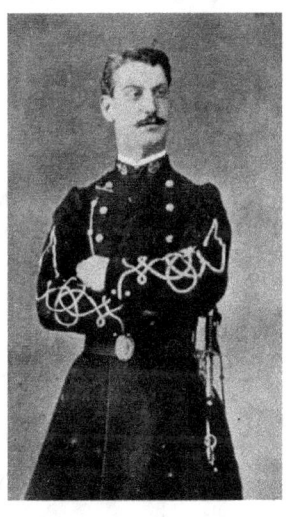

Joseph S. Gallieni
Graduate, Saint-Cyr Academy, 1870
"On the sweet tree of life time
Ripens the bitter fruit of age"
(M. Taillevent, c. 1390-c.1450)

I took office on the 17th of December. The same day, the general confided with my wife, ending with these words: "…The machine starts to wear down and deteriorate. And it just increases my desire to return as soon as possible with younger hands and with the greater vigor I'm used to at my level of function."

Towards the end of December, we had a farewell visit with Dr. Minet[4]. The General received us both in his office. There was a kind of prescient warning of (the General's) short term as Minister. I remember two official portraits adorning the walls of the room: "It is not necessary", he said, "to go on forever with the features I take to do a good job. Look at these portraits: one represents a man who has been in power for two months, the other one who was there for six months, who accomplish the greatest of things. .. I also want to do great things, important reforms, but I must hasten ... Ah! If it weren't for my prostate, I feel I could

---

[4] Emile Henry Minet (1872-1971), French urologist, trained under Felix Guyon and Ernest Desnos at the famed Hôpital Necker

work so well ... Now", he said, turning to me, "it depends on you. Later today I will go over to the President. In three quarters of an hour, my service will be over. My plan has already stopped ... For we must devote ourselves to the task we have undertaken, when there is hardly time to do so. If there were ever a moment that I could just devote to myself more fully, I would simply go away." After we talked a few moments about his vast project, the General then shared with us, rather incidentally, aspects of his life - a method of recall he preferred to do – and that was evidence of the extent of his activities and his concern for all interests, be they ever so humble.

"Here, we must take care of everything. Look, here's a letter from a poor village mayor, complaining that there is no doctor to treat its citizens as they are leaving for the armies from where they had practiced in the country. Well, I'll ask Godart to study the matter and arrange to satisfy this demand, we cannot let these brave people be without medical attention". Thus, at any time, a mark of kindness touched and surprised those who now knew of his true nature rather than the somewhat cold outside of apparent authoritarianism.

On the 30th of December, the General sent for me to ask me about any information on his health. I found him walking, as usual, through his bedroom. He spoke to me, without stopping. "It's boring, you know, to be welded as I am to work. I did not get to relax ... But I had every right to rest ... After Sudan, Tonkin, after Tonkin, Madagascar, after Madagascar, after the Supreme War Council, and then the War ... Just think, the day after the death of my wife – I barely had time for the funeral- I had to return to Paris at once ... And since then, what work! You do not realize it, the Ministry of War touches everything in the country... It was a truth that I was strong to lead such a life, but now it is wrong. And the reality of prostate problems and to be a Minister of War, it does not work together ... So, it is 3 PM. And from 3:30 to 8 PM I will continuously receive senators and deputies, who will speak of their business and waste my time." So, I told the General that he should rest for a few days:

"Obviously, I'd go to St. Raphael to see my tirailleurs[5]: it would do me much good! But it is virtually impossible. I must find another solution for the moment now.'

---

[5] Lit. *riflemen*, a reference to his old infantry battalion, and popular in many of the French Foreign Legions, especially the Regiments of Algerian Tirailleurs who were rushed to defend Paris in 1914.

On January 11th, 1916, at 6:00, the General, between two appointments, took me into his bedroom, very happy to announce that he felt stronger, and indeed, his look was more rested, his complexion clear. It was the first time I had found such improvement. I wanted so much to see the General back that I figured this was a more definitive change. Unfortunately, the duration of these phases was ephemeral, and all in all the bad days outweighed the good. In any case, that day could really be marked with a white stone. It appeared to me that this was probably the result of the change in diet that followed the General. Indeed, trying to fortify the Commander, Charbonnel and I had finally made some improvements in the strict vegetarianism he had practiced for 18 years- 18 years since he had not eaten meat. He flattered himself, moreover, as one of three beneficial resolutions he had made about his health which were: the abolition of meat, abstinence from alcohol, and the adoption of a homoeopathic doctrine. We therefore convinced the General, after a lot of effort, to add to his usual food a little meat and eggs. He took the meat at lunch. As for eggs, he generally consumed them in a kind of raw mix when they were placed in a yellow soup he had in the morning. Thanks to the complicity of the cook, we could make him take two eggs so prepared when he was expecting only one. But fate made him discover the fraud: he growled at the real culprits, but smiling, too.

On the 14th of January at 6:00, the General, running down on his luck, was revisited by the fatigue imposed on him –

"You know," he said, "I'm not happy. You could leave me alone at my age. I paid my debt to the country. After 29 years in the colonies and 15 months in the military government. The least they could do was allow me to rest. They should not have put me into this War, but someone younger."

And stopping suddenly, he turns to me: "Oh! If I could rest at the seaside, sitting on a rock and just think about nothing! Nothing at all!" Then, after a head movement that expresses the disappointment of an unattainable vision, he resumed his walk around his room. I hear his voice from afar: "Mrs. Laval wrote me a kind letter of encouragement ... I am grateful but tell her that I am sad." And then he became silent. We heard only the muffled sounds of his footsteps on the carpet. The word "sad" fell straight as a stone into a bottomless pit. If the General is in fact sad, it would be difficult to realize it, because nothing in his habits betrays any feeling: his alertness, acuity of vision, the energy of his speech, the force of his gestures, none has changed, but inside him there is the disease which, cunningly, exhausts him, thanks

13

to his overwork and struggles for existence. Thus, he feels the progressive difficulty of its course, and he expects that he will not always be able to 'master' it, and a time will come when it will be powerless to hide the failures of his body. Some things cannot be moved! But already the reverberations of this melancholy note are overcome by the incessant preoccupation of the spirit of the Chief. The conversation resumed on a military theme: evolution of the battle, heroism, the conduct of the soldiers, the rapport with our Russian and British allies. The General often thought aloud, until he used his favorite phrase:

"Finally, *voila!*..." which meant that the interview was over.

As I was leaving, he asked me for something for his throat, which was often irritated. With a certain frankness he said to me, "I tried homeopathy which typically works for me but this time I didn't see any effect. Give me one of your allopathic remedies."

After consideration I prescribed a gargle. "Your medication will probably work," he said, "but its effect might not last long. Think about it and find me something else for the day you choose that will make the treatment more effective for me." His prediction was right, as we know, which was further evidence of the General's insight into such things.

Two days later I saw my patient: "Oh, if I could get rid of my prostate, and my relationships with these legislators, he cried, I feel that I could make it to the end of the War..."

Then he added: "The last transactions of the Minister of War. How I would rather be a kid in an amphitheater!"

And he smiled mischievously, his eyes darting from side to me, above his eyeglasses. He seemed happy as a child to see my surprise reaction to his witticism. But the smile quickly fell. The General still felt very tired. He told me he forced himself not to drink almost during the whole day of meetings with the Council of Ministers or the Commission of the Army, in order not to be inconvenienced. Of course, this depletion of drink has other effects most detrimental to his health.

Around the 18th of January I was called by the General to his bedroom. I found him with Dr. Luys, who had come to examine him and made the diagnosis of an enlarged prostate with chronic inflammation of the bladder, the latter of which was to be blamed for most of his observed problems. My colleague believed that local massage[6], with irrigation, would overcome the malady and recover his health.   The General asks for my opinion and I advise him to try the proposed treatment. Accordingly, the new addition of Dr. Luys, at the time mobilized as medical officer of the 2nd class in Besancon, the Military Hospital of Versailles, was decided on the spot. It was agreed that by day Dr. Luys would be assigned to the hospital service and then be on call at night in Paris to continue the care of the Minister.

The first massage took place on Sunday, the 30th of January, at 3 o'clock in the afternoon. The General had chosen that day and hour so as to have the least chance of being disturbed. The treatments, at first, were carried out every two days, following the first visit of

---

[6] Prostatic massage, as once prescribed for prostatitis

16

Dr. Luys[7] and then took place on Tuesday, the 1st of February in the afternoon. We observed the deplorable condition in which the General appeared that day. He had been, in fact, at this session of the Parliament, stormy and rough, when he had to go down to the dais, without being able to be heard. We know the rest: the stupefaction of the deputies, Viviani helping the Minister of War back up to the podium, and then, all deputies gave him a unanimous standing ovation.

I saw him at 7 o'clock, when he returned to the residence. He did not hide his disappointment despite knowing something of parliamentary manners and certainly never suspected the event. And such was his tremendous fatigue, resulting from the exertion for which he was not prepared, he had to undergo his second treatment session. Without doubt, this was an opportunity for physicians to note once again that he had his energy intact, this extraordinary energy that he was to retain until his last breath. He could not, however,

---

[7] Georges Jules Luys (1870-1953), author *Treatise on Cystoscopy and Urethroscopy*, 1918

suppress one complaint:

"Realize that I have issues, of the top importance, to deal with G. Q. G.[8], and to think that I had to lose three hours in the Parliament, this afternoon, with those *mastroquets*[9]! I cannot go on like that...I have to, necessarily, limit myself."

---

[8] 'Grand Quartier General' or General Headquarters

[9] *Mastroquets*, lit. 'wine merchants', used in the derogative

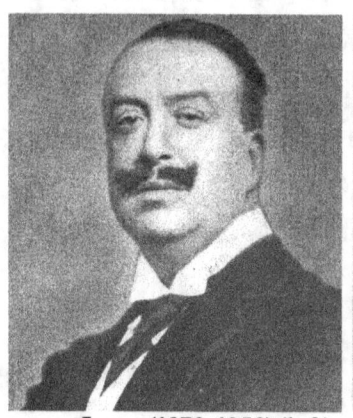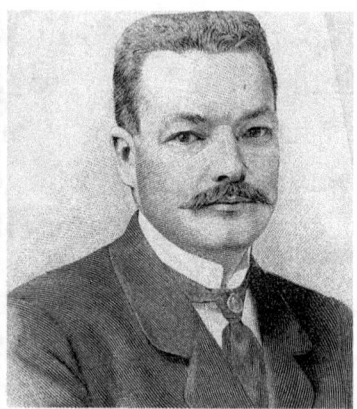

Georges Luys (1870-1953)(left) and J. B. Georges Marion (1869-1960), two of France's greatest urologic surgeons, called to Gallieni's aid in early 1916.

During the days that followed, the General felt his strength diminishing. In a card he wrote on Feb. 6, he jots down "too burdensome " in his opinion, and he adds: "I am being led on-and I doubt I can be led on much longer."

On the 18th of February he had his ninth treatment session, always in the evening at 9:00. The state of things didn't seem so bad.

"I feel better", says the General, at the end of this session. *"Ça va...J'étale"*[10].

At the time, this statement made me very happy. But, on reflection, I remembered having noticed several times already, he often had similar impressions that were never realized, so that, despite everything, I could not help but dread the future.

---

[10] Lit., from *'etaler'*, of a naval derivation, as in 'to resist' or 'withstand a seastroke', figuratively, "I'm all right...I resist."

Then came the tragic day of Verdun and the loss of our troops. Fatigue reappeared in him with worries and sleepless nights. The General had to get up eight or ten times during the night, and his mind stopped working. At the same time, his appetite was poor. We were rapidly losing the ground we had so painfully won. On 25 February, the General said: "What I feel intimidates me, and deprives me of my confidence. And so I need to do something. I just don't know if I can make it until the end."

One can imagine how painful it was to hear him express this conviction, however unfortunately justified, of his not being sure he could hold on until the end.

Given the difficulty of obtaining any substantive improvement, a question arose: was there some stone we were missing, that protracted the troubles suffered by the General? At its simplest, the discovery of a foreign body was almost a desirable thing because a relatively simple operation would have been able to cure the matter. It was therefore appropriate to conduct an exploration to be decisive about this possibility. Dr. Luys and I shared our views with the General, who agreed without much difficulty to consent to a cystoscopy, sustaining our secret hope that perhaps a stone was the cause of all his miseries.

The straight forward exam took place on Saturday, Feb. 26, at 9 o'clock in the evening:

The cystoscopy was negative.

I can still see the General lying on the examination table, in the glare of electric lights in the small white and gold salon, where the procedure was performed, as the procedure came to an end.

He had just learned that we had not found any stone. We could not conceal our disappointment but our silence, however, spoke volumes. I glanced at the corner of the patient's eye, where there was little tear, but his will still upbeat as always.

While smiling, and in his firm, typically loud voice, he says, "Well, too bad!...The only thing now is to just continue treatment!"

He gets up and, gets dressed. We shook hands, then he left us... We deferred the nightly chat we usually had. We felt that he was more tired than usual, and not without reason, too. Those who have had to undergo this kind of exploration by the name cystoscopy, appreciate the amount of energy it must have taken the General to get himself through the ordeal at a night, coming after an exhausting day of labor.

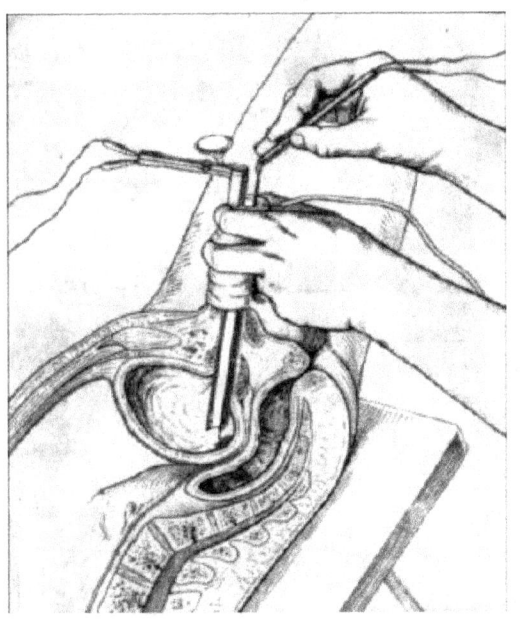

'**Direct' cystoscopy** as illustrated in the 1918 treatise on the subject by Georges Luys, and performed by him on the General in early 1916, the basis of which is that no prism or reflecting lens is used to present an image, a 'direct' view to the examiner. 'Direct' illumination avoided difficulties with early surgical optics but which limited surgical irrigation and instrumentation and was replaced by prism-based or 'indirect' endoscopy as a standard by the1920s.

The next day - Sunday, February 27th, - for the first time, the General had me pay him a house call. The night had been bad. Planting his gaze far into mine, as he did when he raised an important question: "You know," he said, "there is a company known as 'March or Die'. Several of my friends are members. Come, Laval. "Tell me frankly. I'm not a sissy, you know. I must obey the advice and obligations of this society that says to bear with it, to keep on walking without rest, without hesitation? Or, should I retire, resign my position to rest and take care of myself? Do not be afraid to hurt me. I want to know."

I thought for a moment. The conflict that reigned in the soul of the General was like the one he had just awakened in me. What advice was there to give? So many different elements and such important things were rattling in my mind that I hesitated to answer. In reality, the question posed to me could be reduced to the simple formula: was there no hope that the General could keep going, to continue his lifestyle, and pursue the current treatments? Or, rather, could a cure be expected without resorting to rest or other means? I finally

25

responded that in my mind, one could wait for at least a few days, pending any other additional improvements. The General did not reply and thus accepted my advice. But he thought for a moment and, in a kind of conclusion of his thoughts, he could not help but tell me, with is customarily ironic air:

"Life's fun, is it not?" In these simple words, without further recrimination, I guessed what he had suffered and what he should suffer yet: intimate sorrow, loss of a beloved wife, away from his children and grandchildren; the disappointed soul of a soldier; his health making him unable to travel to his troops, in particular, to go to Verdun, which played the largest part of the War since the Battle of the Marne, a surrender of his best hope, of ever again commanding again against the enemy. And finally his progressive collapse, being plagued by an evil against which the fight was becoming harder and harder...

On the 3rd of March, the General said: "I'll try to finish the job imposed upon me by High Command, and then I think it would be better to go away because this time I'm really exhausted. I can do no more..." And he added: "Ah! It is just simply not convenient to go, and address issues like this in the state of health I'm in now".   Undoubtedly the situation worsened, the weakness increased, and the General sometimes was unsteady walking. He tried to recover, deploying an almost superhuman energy, but, alas! in vain, there was no concealing it. It became obvious he could not continue his duties. But as it was a decision to make, whose scope exceeds that of the individual, a consultation was considered necessary.

It took place March 5th in the bedroom of the General: the consultant was Dr. Marion. His opinion, which concurred with that of Dr. Luys and mine, was explicit: first, an urgent need for complete rest for one month away from Paris – to Versailles, for example, where Dr Marion was attached to the Military Hospital there and could continue to see the patient. It was understood, moreover, that the rest would allow him "to follow proper treatment, to undergo, if any, intervention, and in any case, to resume active service within about two months" (From the notes of the consultation).

"Well, that's it then!" concluded the General. "I relegate myself into your hands. You will try to get me back on my feet. If you do, I will present myself to the Government a cured man, and can go anywhere, in short, will be able to lead a life like everyone else.

"I am at your disposition, I would say to the President of the Republic; do with me what you want...Otherwise, I know that my role is done and we wouldn't talk any more about it ... I so would have liked to command as well and die on the front ..." And, while the General uttered these last words, his voice seemed weaker than usual, but his eyes shone with an unusual splendor.

When we left, it was understood that he would read the next day, to the Council of Ministers, his report on the reorganization of the High Command, and subsequently that the task he had set upon would be finished; he would ask to resign from the government for health reasons.

The 6th of March was painful and cumbersome. We felt back "at the home front" that something serious was brewing. I was questioned on all sides and, of course, I could not answer. On the morning of March 7, as he had expected, the General read his report to the Council of Ministers, then at 5:00 in the evening, in the presence of the President of the Republic, he handed in his resignation to the Chairman, Mr. Briand. The latter, before accepting the resignation, asked the General to reconsider over the next forty-eight hours.

During the afternoon, Commander Charbonnel went with me to Versailles to visit a furnished apartment belonging to long-standing family friends of the Gallieni's, a Mrs. and Miss Adam, who had retained a room at the Hotel des Reservoirs. This apartment offered in response to a request by the General, was immediately accepted by all of us.

On the 8th and 9th of March, all at the Ministry of War existed in an anxious wait, as conflicting versions circulating about the Government's intentions. As for the General, he was calm as usual, but, as usual, he slept badly. When I saw him at 9 in the morning:

"Imagine," he said smiling, "I dreamed of Painlevé[11] and his questions (Mr. Painlevé had visited him the day before). Ah! My mind is tired! I wonder if it will ever recover."

---

[11] Paul Painlevé (1863-1933), French Cabinet member under Aristide Briand, 1915

We made it to March 10th. Three days ago the government received the resignation of General, and we were still awaiting their timely response. As for him, 'a cat is a cat', and a resolution is something that we do not go back on: he has informed the President that he intends to leave the Department the same day, at 4 o'clock. And, indeed, as 4 o'clock struck, the start of the events took place, simple, but beautiful and dignified.

The General appeared in his sky blue uniform and, as usual, impassive and his own master. However, for those who knew him, he was a little worked up and his face was even paler than it was in recent days. He gets into the car which was waiting at the bottom of the stairs, followed by Commander Charbonnel. As the car turns and goes through the court, the civil guards presented arms, as they do each time the Minister comes out, no more, no less.

There was no farewell, since the General was still Minister of War. A number of officers, who had watched the Cabinet initially behind the windows of the entrance hall to the left, were present in silence as this scene unfolded and they experience a certain feeling of anxiety, it seemed, like a dark cloud obscured the skies of France. For the General was beloved, revered, and from those who saw this could not help thinking that it was a permanent departure. And then, what would happen? The Battle of Verdun continued, the country was concerned, and the Government was trying to conceal its apprehensions. What a situation for France to be in such a private moment of a leader who had all the most unwavering confidence!

II

In Versailles

———————

The apartment located in the Hôtel des Réservoirs was on the first floor to the left - seen from outside - and above the front door, with every window facing the street.

Next to the bedroom of the General, was a large living room where he spent his days and took his meals prepared by his cook, whom he had brought with him, in order to continue his special diet. Commander Charbonnel and I had to share his table.

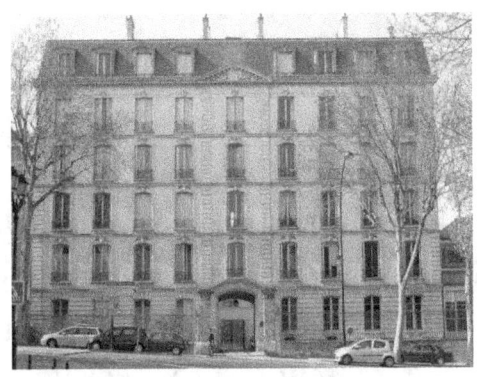

Hôtel des Réservoirs, Versailles, Gallieni's refuge from Paris while awaiting his first of two prostate surgeries. Adjacent to the verdant gardens of Versailles, the residence was built by Louis XV for his mistress Madame Pompadour. Enlarged copiously in the 1900's, it served as a resort hotel, housing Marcel Proust for a month, and later the German delegation who arrived to sign the Treaty of Versailles in 1919.

From the day after our arrival, as his cough had increased somewhat, the General had to keep to his room. This seclusion did not prevent him to experience a soothing sense of relaxation.

"I feel better already," he said. In his desire to create within and around him an atmosphere of calm to reach his goal more quickly, he began to form heroic resolutions so he did not want to read newspapers, hear about the government, or even to keep abreast of the events of the war. He no longer intended to receive any visits outside the Executive Cabinet's Colonel Bouccabeille, who would present the more urgent daily business of his department.

In an attempt to appease his spirit, and occupy his mind swirling with thoughts, he immersed himself in books.

While reading very quickly and with much attention, there was in him such a ferment of ideas that in his reading, some comment or remarks would suddenly escape from him and we would ask a question quite independent of his subject, and he would always demonstrate an extraordinary keenness of mind.

"I feel the cold outside," he told me one day, "but under this head there is a such a tempest. I think all the time, day and night... alas!" He could not help be distracted by his thoughts not only when reading, but sometimes also, I believe, whenever they occurred.

After reading for a while, often quite long, he would get up, hands in the pockets of his jacket, according to his familiar attitude, that attitude that has so captivated his eminent sculptor, Maillard[12] - he walked into the living room, firm and deliberate, speaking of everything from newspaper articles that he could no longer read - the Government - which he had promised not to think about - and war – with which he was no longer occupied... and also concern for the colonies, Madagascar, in particular, his travels, to his childhood memories; medicine, homeopathy, which was above all, his favorite subject.

His memory was wonderfully faithful.

---

[12] Auguste Maillard, (1864-1944) was later commissioned to create a bronze medallion bearing Gallieni's likeness, sold from July, 1916 "for the national benefit" and which placed on Gallieni's tomb at St. Rafaël.

One example among many: in the conversations telling me about his captivity in 1870, he said without hesitation the name of his orderly, his German teacher, people he had gotten to know in the small Bavarian town where he was a prisoner. He never forgot a proper name, never a word or turn of phrase- always recalling them at the first shot, and they just flowed without any effort. And the accuracy of his memory, and the sharpness of his elocution, these he retained until his death.

I used the period of calm we went through to try to raise the condition of the patient through subcutaneous injections, tonics and stimulants. But he was still not free of the burden of his ministerial duties, Admiral Lacaze, Minister of the Navy, being responsible only for the interim of the war, that is to say the workings of current affairs - and again, officially only since March 14. This situation was not without concern to the General, and he did not feel free from all worries.

Finally, on March 16th, he learned that the Government had decided to appoint a successor, General Roques. Then, on the morning of the 16th, General Gallieni drew up his letter of resignation, newspapers published that Commander Charbonnel would soon be President of the Council in Paris.

This question now settled, the General's burden was immediately reduced.

"It's funny, I really feel ready to start something else. I think of what I shall do when I am restored to health."

The responsibilities, despite his departure from the department, that he had felt he ceased to perform, still prevented him from fully enjoying the change of his environment, but the next day was better than previous ones. And this improvement appeared promising.

On the 19th, in fact, there was an increase in weight; the general's mood improved, and his usual playfulness, which, for some time, had darkened, became once more cheerful: he recovered the ability to joke.

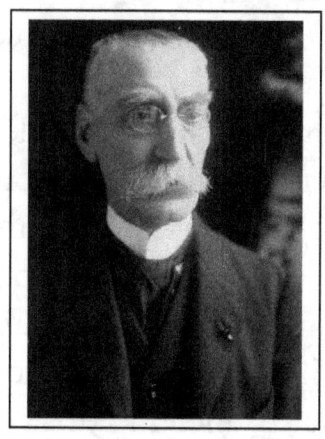

Joseph S. Gallieni (1849-1916)
Minister of War, in civilian clothes, December, 2015.
National Library of France

Nevertheless, despite these assumptions, the desired outcome was delayed. On March 21st, the General found that "(he wasn't) improving fast enough" and how boring it was to have an "empty brain."

"It worked so hard, my brain!" he noted… "Me, when I have an idea in mind, it doesn't let go until it is completed. Until then I'm always in anguish. And then, once finished, other ideas take the place of newly conceived ones, and so on ... You see it from here. .. That's the way it is…and it is not very restful."

He had a decreased appetite. From the first bite of food, the General was no longer hungry, his tongue was overwhelmed, he was very tired and sometimes at night, a little feverish.

It was in those circumstances, that on April 2nd, Dr. Marion took over management of the treatment. The plan of the surgeon was: to let the body fully rest up and, once there was a sufficient amount of improvement, perform an operative prostatectomy in two stages, the second being undertaken only when the local situation and his general condition were good enough to optimize the chances of success of the more challenging stage. At the same time, in addition, Dr. Marion offered to get a second opinion for the General, if he so desired, for further advice on the most correct course of action. But the General declined the offer and said he was fully confident in the treatment offered by Dr. Marion as much as he was in the person who proposed it.

The night of April 2nd to 3rd was one of the most relaxing that General had had in a long time. A significant improvement was appreciated that could be seen in his face.

The cough had almost ceased, the weather helped, and he began daily jaunts out in the *Parc du Chateau*[13]. The first took place on April 3. The General, flanked by his aide and his doctor, began his walk around 11 o'clock. The park, already decorated with foliage of spring, was almost empty. We did meet some strollers, however, who, alerted by our uniforms, recognized the General's characteristic silhouette snug in his little black coat, cinched in at the waist: they greeted him with reverence.

Was he not the Savior of their city? He replied with his usual good spirits, without interrupting his conversation. He accepted all these natural displays of reverence, but never thought to draw the slightest sense of pride from them.

---

[13] The large tracts of gardens and paths that surrounded the Palace at Versailles, including the Gardens and Orangerie, built for Louis XIV in the 1660s by, among others Jules Hardouin-Mansart.

This first outing lasted just twenty minutes. The figure of twenty minutes might be surprising. It was thus so with the General, whose clear mind so appreciated such things, especially its clarity and precision, that it was essential to determine in advance the duration of the walk. And unless special events determined otherwise this objective should be and had been observed.

Walks took place then, every day, a little longer each time and never exceeding forty minutes. They were little noticed. No photographers or reporters: the General abhorred anything that could give rise to the idea of advertising.

Eschewing popularity and finding tasteful only that narrow circle of those whom he loved, he received no one, apart from his own and a few visitors, such as General Weick, his discreet and devoted friend, Colonel Vallieres, his former fellow prisoner in Sudan, who often came to inquire after him on behalf of the President of the Republic, Mr. Justin Godant, then Sub-Secretary Secretary of State, Department of Health, whom he had known formerly in Lyons and showed great cordiality. A friendly visit that touched many was that of Lord Kitchener. Called to the mission in Paris, he had asked to be received by the General. Despite the fatigue that inevitably would result from such a meeting, it was impossible not to yield to the wishes of the British Minister because of those particular bonds of sympathy that so united him with General Gallieni. The visit took place so without any pomp, in the most noble simplicity, in complete privacy, and when at the end of this conversation, which lasted nearly an hour, Commander Charbonnel and I were called in to witness the departure of Lord Kitchener. I had the impression of seeing two great men separated as two friends, honest and sincere, in a fair handshake, just to say a "goodbye". In reality, the handshake was a seal on their ultimate farewell. These hcrocs, outwardly so robust, were both soon to disappear, each one in a way as abrupt and unexpected as the other. When, after the departure of Lord Kitchener, I saw the General, he could not help tell me:

"With him, we understand, we walk hand in hand, '*the hand in the hand*'," he repeated in English (because he spoke fluent English).

The only official visits were when the General received Mr. Poincare, the President of the Republic, a few visits from Admiral Lacaze, and during a respite, as he was assured, the last visit of General Roques, who at the time took care of the war papers.

This almost monastic life of the General could not fail to arouse curiosity and cause all sorts of gossip and suppositions. Whenever some enquired about him, as the nosey often could about his private life, he smiled, then shrugged his shoulders. One day, about an event in which he was alleged to be the hero:

"If you were in the situation I am in now, you'd avoid such stupid chatter, " he said in a mocking tone. Other "gossip" circulated just as absurd as it always arises when concerning great men. "The General", it was said, "wants to have surgery to get married then with Mrs. X."

One of my friends, and a distinguished physician, one of the best known in Paris, asked me if it was true that General was "a rabid smoker of opium." Another said: "Is it true that he has inoperable cancer of the prostate?"

The following story is worth telling.

Several people confided to me that everyone knew the inclination of General to Madame Z. and that the lady then showed sympathy towards him. Some cited as proof of the fact that, upon his arrival to Versailles, the General had found on his table a beautiful bouquet, a delicate attention Mrs. Z. had placed there. Although it was true that a bouquet was laid on the table of the General, Commander Charbonnel and I were in a better position than anyone to know which friends could have provided such a friendly gesture.

Other rumors were circulated later, otherwise serious and somewhat hard to deal with because, as we know, there are now still some people who are indeed doubting the actual conditions of the death of General Gallieni.

We will return to that later.

Nevertheless, the General kept thinking of the events unfolding on the Verdun front and he could not help making the forecasts that he said, took into account what was going on: he provided such insights as was a part of his nature. While walking in his living room - because he refrained from discussing the war - he decided:

"Now is the time to do this, to prepare for it... If you wait, it will be too late ..."

And he criticized the spirit of optimism which continued to prevail in the inner circles which was necessary, in his view, to see the realities in their true light.

His general condition had improved enough by April 7th and the following assessment of his health was written:

"After a slight fall six days ago, the General's condition was still serious. Appetite better, sleep has returned the past few days - for the first time in two months - was able to go out for short trips on foot in the park every day. The General has found it going quite well. In short, the situation has improved significantly, and, better still, if it were at all feasible, that the operation would be carried out within a fortnight. "

These objectives were realized, and the date of the first intervention was determined: the 20th of April.

The day before the selected date, at 4 o'clock, the General, accompanied by his children, by Mrs. Gruss and by Lieutenant Gallieni, who had come home from the Belgian front, all came to the Hospital of the Augustinian Sisters at 27 Rue Maurepas - which operated at the same time an auxiliary Hospital Auxiliary of the French Ladies Association. He came to occupy the left part of the facility available in the home, a modest room in the Annex, at its end, as far as possible from the comforts of home: an iron-framed bed in the middle, a dresser, a wardrobe, a dressing table and some chairs were the only furniture, but furniture that was clear, white, very clean and smartly arranged; the adjoining room was used as a parlor for pets and for the General to take his meals when he would be able to get up.

On Thursday, the 20th of April, I arrived at the Hospital at 7:15. I found that the General had arranged everything: the night had been exceptionally good. It would have been impossible to detect in him the slightest trace of emotion: the pulse was slow and in its customary regularity. Once he was dressed, he was ready to descend to the operating room:

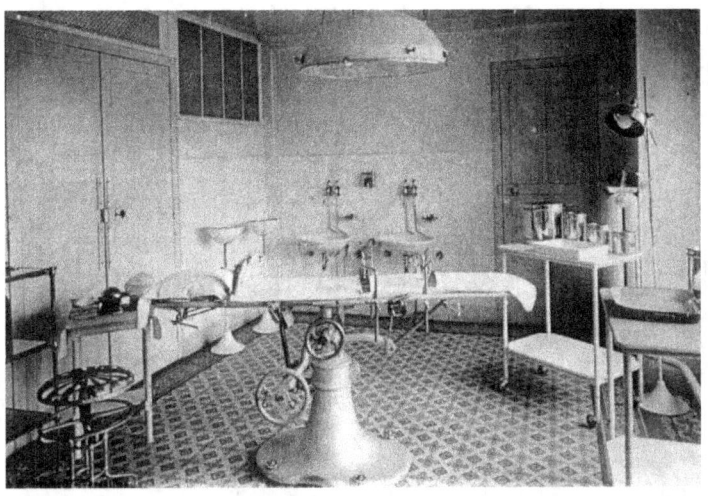

Operating room, Clinique Franciscan, Versailles, 1930s, typical of the era where, in 1916, Gallieni underwent two surgeries, the first, under local, to place a suprapubic tube and the second, general anesthesia, the prostatectomy.

"Then, let's go to the sacrifice!" he said to me smiling. "But I hope," he added, "that I will return here on foot."

"Forget it, sir," I replied, "That is quite impossible."

"But why not? Marchand, who is also a soldier, managed quite well when entering the hospital. He didn't make it through to the end, it's true, but it's still just a few steps."

"My General, there will be a wound and, when you return, any movements you make could rupture the stitches there."

He made that head movement which always meant: "So be it!" but, as we will see later, he did not consider himself beaten.

The intervention - the cystostomy – was carried out under local anesthesia with cocaine. The General bore it with his usual composure, even joked at times. "What a pity that the operation did not occur in front of the troops!" exclaimed Dr Marion as he removed his hand from placing the last stitch. "What a fine example you would have given them!" "They do not need it", the General remarked quite simply.

Then he immediately replied:

"But I really hope you'll let me walk back to my room". That was basically because he did not want to come back on a stretcher. Dr. Marion and I had a lot of trouble in convincing him that to avoid problems that sometimes result from the use of cocaine, and that he could potentially sever the edges of the wound altogether, that he absolutely needed to be brought back in the supine position.

But once settled into his bed, the General returned to this subject and the bitter disappointment he experienced.

"Did you suffer much, father?" asked Mrs. Gruss.

"Ah, yes, a little," the General evasively replied. "But what bothered me the most was to be transported on a stretcher and to see those kids watch me as I passed by! ..."

He was referring to the young people who had watched curiously in the passageway, when he had gone downstairs, and who did not fail to show up in the hallway to see him again we he returned. To have given this show for an "operation so small," as he had considered the cystostomy, had generated in him a feeling of humiliation that was very painful.

When Dr. Marion came to greet him before his departure:

"Well, Doctor," said the Chief with an evil eye, "it hasn't gone too badly, this small battle in the outpost?"

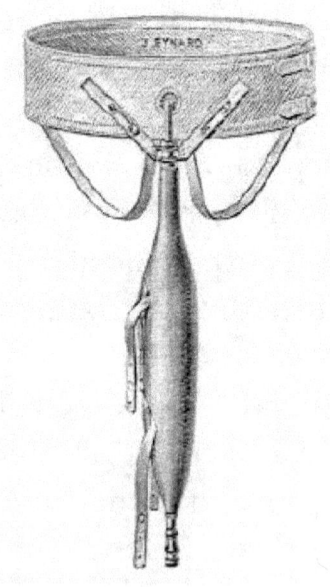

"Apparatus of Professor Marion for Cystostomy". Early urinary cystostomy catheters could dislodge so the above device was used by Marion and others to secure suprapubic urinary tubes, and would allow patients, like Gallieni, to walk with less fear of tube dislodgement (from J. Eynard & Cie, Urology)

In the days following the surgery he received many expressions of sympathy. One of those he found most touching was a shipment of lemons, with a card bearing the words:

"Two Americans, great friends of France, send to the Savior of Paris, the brave General Gallieni, with their wishes for a speedy recovery, picked these lemons to calm the fever that always follows operations. And until his recovery, he will receive these fresh munitions".

In fact, shipments of lemons regularly followed.

As would be expect, the General found himself feeling tired during the first days, but after April 25, that is to say, the 6th post-operative day – he began to stand and sit in the little room adjoining his bedroom.

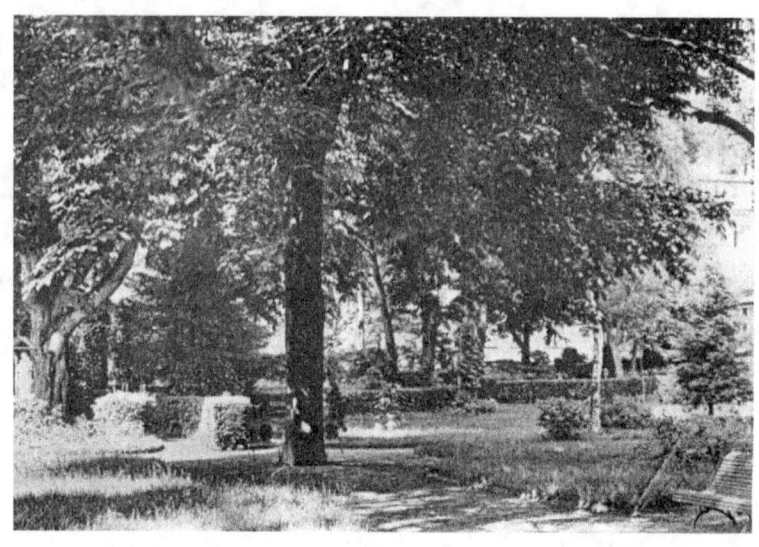

Garden behind the Clinique Franciscaine, Versailles, 1930s. Here, Gallieni would stroll after his first operation, just a few steps or minutes, but in the pleasant climate of spring, 1916. H. Bessard, Yvelline Archives, Versailles.

On the 27th he made his first outing in the hospital garden. The days, rather dull until then, had become quite beautiful: the sun shone brightly that morning. Around 4 o'clock the General was set down onto a sedan chair and placed between two hedgerows, where he was sheltered from the wind, and had plenty of light.

Delighted, he bore very well that first encounter with the outdoors for about an hour.

Thereafter, almost every day he spent time in the garden. Getting outside was giving him much pleasure, because, through the exercise resulting from walking, he felt his strength revive.

Clad in his pajamas, purple jacket, and sky blue trousers, a cap of the same color adding style to the energetic leader, his hand resting on a solid cane of Madagascar applewood[14], the General made a number of garden tours, then rested on his chair, then, before returning to his room, completed the number of laps that had been predetermined. The place where he stopped varied with the days: when it was sunny and warm, it was in a hedgerow lined with relatively

---

[14] "Pomme d'argent"

dense shrubs; if the air was a bit cold, we would move within the wall of the garden, surrounded by a strawberry patch; if it rained, in the greenhouse. At 4:00, the faithful Bouvier, an orderly of the General –who had been injured in the war - brought him something tasty usually composed of a cup of chocolate milk, drank it with a straw, and two croissants split in the middle and toasted; sometimes he also accepted some fruit.   During the walks the General kept talking. At rest, he still spoke or read but it was very rare that he remained immersed in thought. They talked about everything except art, which didn't interest him much. He recited with confidence and a remarkable memory passages from the *Iliad* and the *Odyssey*, passed without transition to poems of Lord Baron, then to scenes of Wallenstein, and verses by Goethe. He loved to talk about Madagascar and the administrative organization that was established there. He discussed questions of colonialism with utmost attention, when I was alone with him, and with those who were most interested. One day he was busy describing to me an example of the support and important roles played by French doctors at consular posts in China, when he was interrupted by the arrival of an officer who came from Paris. He was updated with new military details and they talked together for more than twenty minutes on the war situation. The general could not help but see himself as still responsible defending his country, and eventually jumped: "How is it that we do not do this? How are we not prepared for it? ... Ah! if only it weren't for my prostate!" he cried at last with a gesture of annoyance.

At the end of that conversation when the officer had left, the General turned to me and in a most simple way, without hesitation, he went back to his story to the exact spot where he had several moments before had left off.

"Well, the doctor of the consular post of which I spoke enjoyed such a reputation among the Chinese people that he was asked to see the wife of Taô-Taï (whom men were never allowed to see) and that when we went with him into the city, they had fireworks there in his honor, paper dragons, in short, all those festivities one would expect of any kind befitting a victorious commander. Now you see what may be the moral influence of the doctor in the colonies?"

It was during these talks he explained to me his plan of an official Health Service during the war, when, as he hoped, he would resume his active duties.

"I wish," he said, "that all progress made by the Health Department during this campaign was studied and the subject of reports. There would be reports provided to committees composed of prominent figures, professors, academics, etc..., who would look after each study of the major issues in medicine, surgery, epidemiology, hygiene, and many would prepare reports on what has been done during the war...Consider what I say ..." In the garden, the wounded or sick military civilians would pause and salute the General, pointing out the curiosity to their parents or friends. He responded with a frank smile, sometimes he addressed them with a few simple words from the heart and of such a kind as he knew how to speak, walk and then resume his normal conversation.

At 5:00 sharp, earlier if the weather was cool or if fatigue set in, the general would get back to his bedroom.

And at the Hotel des Reservoirs he received very few visits, those of his children and especially his grandchildren were particularly pleasing. Robert and Lucienne, who were very wise despite their young age, provoked the admiration of their grandfather. We felt very happy to see the development of young minds. After having held them for just a few moments in his arms and peppered them with a question or two, he embraced them, and then they withdrew in order not to tire.

After a fortnight, the patient's general condition had improved notably, the temperature did not exceed normal, and his appetite was sufficient, and what was especially desirable was that the extreme thinness of his overall appearance gave way to an appearance of plumpness, his strength returned, and the General could walk without wobbling, which he had not been able to do for a long time, and, finally, the examination of urea in the blood and a renal permeability test using methylene blue had both given satisfactory results. Under these conditions, it was logical to consider the more crucial operation. However, Dr. Marion made sure to discuss with the General beforehand, if he preferred to stay in the state it was, rather than run the chances of a new intervention. But the General did not wish to stop along the way.

"No", he replied. "It's all or nothing.[15]
"From here on out, if I were to live with this disability which now impairs me and always be so reliant on continued treatments, I would be good for nothing. I would just have to be locked

---

[15] *"C'est tout ou rien."*

up at home. I must admit, if I could resume some service, nothing could hinder me."

In view of this statement and given the favorable conditions in which the General was now in, it was decided that the second surgery would take place on Thursday, May 18th, that is to say twenty-eight days after the first.

Gradually, the appointed day arrived, and not without some apprehension on my part, and certainly also with regard to Dr. Marion. We recognized the great esteem to which we held our patient, and we were not unaware of the hopes founded on his return to health, but we were certain that he would achieve a full recovery, even earlier than expected. How, indeed, could there be such circumstances as to not undergo the desired surgical procedure? The failure of this attempt could have such consequences for the country, that we dared to consider the proposition of success[16]. The most careful precautions were taken to leave nothing to chance: we even prepared for the religious habits of the General, had it been necessary.

To minimize the serial causes of fatigue, it was

---

[16] "*hypothèse*", here, the sense of presumption or possibility.

agreed that the patient would be put to sleep using ethyl chloride given by successive inhaled doses, and that the anesthesia would be extended if necessary by a few drops of chloroform, according to the process known as 'chloroform to the Queen.'[17] For his part, the surgeon would act with the utmost rapidity.

The general appeared "to submit" to the whole affair, in good spirits. The prostatectomy operation began at 8 am, Dr. Marion was assisted by Dr. Friteau and Madamoiselle Dr. Kogan; I was responsible for general anesthesia. This was achieved through two successive doses of 5 cc of ethyl chloride, then a couple of drops of chloroform. Although the prostate was large and difficult to remove, everything was finished and in excellent shape about 8:15, that is to say, about a quarter of an hour after the start. The organ was extracted in full and embodied what would be typically called a simple adenoma.

---

[17] *"chloroforme à la reine"*, a reference to the anesthesiologic method used effectively by John Snow, in 1853, on Queen Victoria during the birth of her son, Crown Prince Leopold.

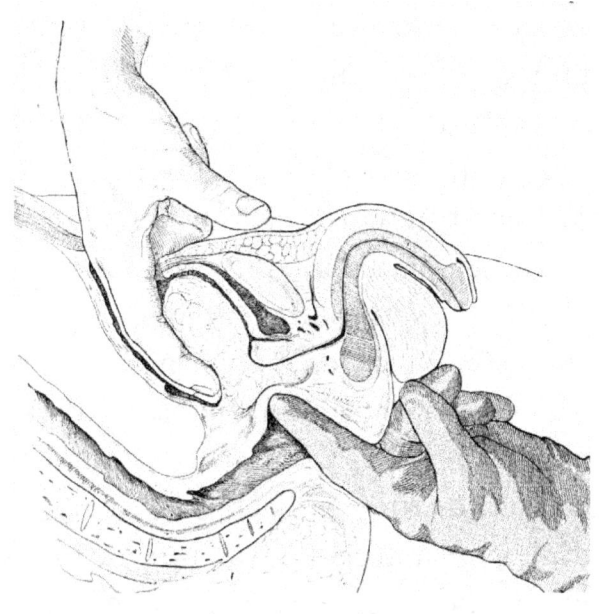

Suprapubic Prostatectomy, from *Treatise on Urology,* 1921. By Georges J. B. Marion. The procedure, using the gloved hand to push the prostatic adenoma towards the ungloved operator finger was said to take, in Gallieni's case and performed by Marion himself, 15 minutes.

Once back in bed, the General, who had hitherto remained almost unconscious, sustained his first bouts of significant discomfort. These, fortunately, did not last. Throughout the rest of the day, the patient recovered somewhat, and brightened up. But as Mr. Gheusi has noted in his book, *War and Theater,* immobility is problematic: "(Immobility) affected his greatest hours of convalescence after he separated (from the troops) and left for St. Raphaël. And this means more to him than most think: the fighting that continues around the Douaumont is his greater concern, and he makes them repeat the details."

The night was pretty good, and the General rested. After he experienced at first some reluctance to drink, he eventually overcame the disgust and began to take in liquids. His spirits were always excellent. The aftermath of the operation itself appeared absolutely normal until the 21st of May, when a complication occurred which suddenly brought about a gloomy prognosis. That morning, when the packing left in place at the end of the operation had been removed by the surgeon himself, profuse bleeding developed about a half an hour later. This prompted the urgent call for Dr. Marion, who rushed back immediately. But despite the speed with which appropriate care was given, the General's condition had suddenly worsened: the skin became very pale, the pulse bad. From here, I ask permission to copy from my notes.

"... May 21st, 2100 hours. - Malfunction of the kidneys in the afternoon, then vomiting of blood with a few clots, towards evening. At night, the urine eventually returned. But the General is in shock, pulse small, irregular. Alas, I fear it is lost. We fight back with serum, camphor oil, caffeine, sparteine[18] ... but there's no effect or just so little!

"May 22, 10:00. Yesterday, after I left the General after midnight, and while he did not look very strong, there seemed to be trend for an improvement. And it was in this morning that I did see a marked improvement, pulse more regular, albeit weak, there was abundant urine.

When dressing, the General joked:

---

[18] Derived from *Scoparius*, and related to digitalis, sparteine was first studied by Mills in 1863 and Fick in 1870 for its effect on cardiac dysrhythmias.

"Finally," he says, "if I go, I will at least have the consolation of going away without my prostate." But he hopes not to go, he has full confidence in his fate, and I had at the time a similar conviction.

"May 23, 9:00 am. - The General is a bit down, sleepy, speaking little but always an energetic face and bright eyes when he opens them. He did not drink all night.

Copious sputum, constant nausea. By really exerting himself this morning, he started to take in some milk.

For a moment he feels oppressed: he is given oxygen to breathe, to great relief.

He is still interested in the battle of Verdun and occasionally raises questions about the general situation.

Dr. Mark, who once treated him with great success and whom was asked to provide a consultation, prescribed a homeopathic potion to be applied with a local compress. He considered it a desperate situation. From some visitors, I learned that in Paris sinister rumors circulated about the General at this point. Surprisingly, in some circles, it was said he was shot to death by a pistol fired by a discontented general, during a discussion.

The hemorrhage that occurred on the 21st of May, as reported by the newspapers, seem to have a certain consistency with this ridiculous fable. I went to bed sad, rooted as I was in my belief that the General would not recover. . . "

The 24th was a bad day. The General, whose stomach could not tolerate even small quantities of liquid, had cool extremities, a very feeble pulse, his eyes were less clear and his complexion had become an almost pale gray. In addition, he spoke little, and tried to "conserve" his breaths most of the time.

Dr. Parmentier, physician at the Hôpital Saint-Antoine, was called in for a consultation: he felt that due to his very poor stomach tolerance and the patient's insurmountable distaste for food, he could not be fed by mouth. Instead, he advocated artificial feeding, copious injections of glucose at the same time as stimulants: caffeine, sparteine, camphor oil.

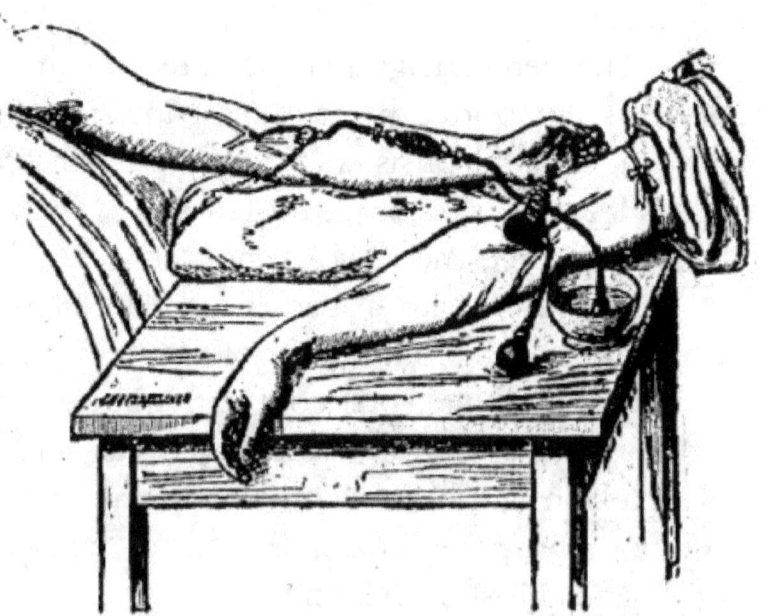

Direct Tranfusion from living donor to recipient, as above in 1880, had been attempted years before knowledge of blood group antigens. As in Gallieni's case, with Dr. Marion as the donor, immediate rejection would be expected in 2 of 3 cases. (from Roussel. *Transfusion Directed du Sang Vivant.* 1883)

Obediently, without any recrimination, the General accepted these treatments. (The General) combined all his efforts with ours; all his energy concentrated in the ardent desire for healing, which will endure from him until his last moments. From time to time, a brief call, he loves the military terminology, he requests oxygen: - *Obus*[19] ...

And he draws in long breaths, quickly, of this vital gas, as to force it to incorporate its substance and revitalize his exhausted state.

Under the influence of all these medications the best day was the 25th. The pulse was stronger, the extremities warmed. Dr. Parmentier returned to see the patient in the morning. He was of the opinion that we should continue to give nothing by mouth, but only towards the end of the day, so that perhaps the patient could try to absorb something from a little hot tea. Furthermore, we plan, without talking to General, the possibility of an attempted transfusion of blood the next day, if the long-awaited improvement was not seen.

---

[19] "*Obus*", a kind of military shell or bomb is, here, a reference to a metal tank of oxygen

In the evening, the General was presented with a cup of chamomile tea: for nearly 40 hours he had had nothing to drink. As the nursed held the cup to his lips, he turned his head, raising both hands and then quietly placed them on the bed, on either side of him, a gesture of an order.

"Let me…direct…the movement, " he said in a low and somewhat breathless voice.

Always the leader who commands! But this time oh how poor you are!

No sooner does he take in a few teaspoons of tea that he can not continue due to severe stomach pains.

The oppression increases.

"But my heart goes!" he told me looking straight at me.

I gave him a few breathes of oxygen and that gave him some relief.

The night of May 25th to 26th was poor. At midnight he had a calming injection to alleviate the suffering; a half hour later, sleep came, and he was able to be so the rest of the night.

On the morning of the 26th, as we had agreed to do if the situation did not become clear, we proposed to the General to try a transfusion of blood. He accepted without any difficulty, having resolved to do anything to try to regain the strength he felt was increasingly abandoning him.

The procedure took place about 10 o'clock.

Having secured the transfusion needle in the vein of the General, Dr Marion offered his own arm for the scalpel, which was administered by Dr. Parmentier. I handled the (transfusion) device. About 150 grams of venous blood were injected into the General. It all went well, very calmly, and during the procedure he experienced no discomfort. As often occurs in such cases, the immediate aftermath of the transfusion was felt: the patient was agitated, his pulse very small, his extremities had become purplish and very cold, and, in short, life seemed to withdraw.

Around 5 o'clock, after a short sleep caused by a soothing injection, the General asked for a drink and, to our surprise, he who, in recent days, could not absorb liquids by teaspoon, began to drink several sips directly from a glass of water mixed with raspberry syrup.

The limbs then regained their normal color and warmth returned, and his breathing less labored, signs which had lost their appearance. In the presence of such a change against all odds, the hope of those in the General's entourage was restored. But the weakness continued.

A little before midnight the patient complained:

"It can not last long, call Laval!" he exclaimed.

I found myself in the next room and I jumped up, charged by the timbre of the General's voice. As soon as I saw the patient's pale face, almost bloodless, his gaze distant as it was full, his breathing short and choppy, I realized that the words he had uttered would probably be the last.

And indeed, the agony began, a short period of suffering in silence. Like when he commanded the room itself to receive the care his entourage gave him, he seemed to say to Death: "One moment. . . not so quickly. . . I'm ready. . ."

Midnight arrived when, surrounded by his children and his sister, Mrs. Martin, General Gallieni breathed his last, simply, nobly, sitting straight up, his eyes wide open, a Chief who knows neither fear nor blame.

A bat flew in hitting the walls and ceiling of the small room which ended the beautiful and serene moment. When the *bird of night*[20] was seen flying out into the evening air through the half opened window, the soul of the General had also gone.

And now – the 27th of May, at 9:00 am – the General is at rest on his bed in his sky blue uniform, adorned with the Military Medal and Croix de Guerre - the only two decorations he wore habitually – to which was added his medallion of the Grand Cross of the Legion of Honor.

---

[20] "l'oiseau des nuits"

His family mourned in silence with him ...

Many visitors filed past the body. Soldiers came there to kneel. Amidst their tears, the sister of the General whispers in my ear:

"He loved them so much, the soldiers! His father repeated all the time: 'The soldier above all. Remember that in difficult circumstances, we must sacrifice everything to the soldier...'

Our father gave him further advice when he was a battalion commander. My poor late brother listened with great respect, then taking me aside, I clarified: 'Would you believe that Dad thinks that I am still a child? But you must listen, there's always something to learn in what a father says...' "

And it is such sweet and tender memories, mixed with the agonizing pain of the loss of a loved one, which the vigilant guard raises up as the glory of death, from the cities and out into the countryside, as it was for the Army, France mourns the loss of one of its best soldiers, one on which she based so much hope in the gloomy hours while he lived...

III

CONCLUSION

If you want to identify the real causes of the death of General Gallieni, we must, in my view, look not so much in the aftermath of the operations, but in the particularly difficult circumstances with which he found himself taken from his position.

I recalled the first bout of retention which occurred in April 1914. Following this incident without immediate aftermath, his normal life resumed, and the General had every intention of living out his days until he retired at Saint Raphaël , *enfin*!

If nothing had gotten in the way, and he had been able to live well on his property, lead a quiet existence, dieting, taking, as appropriate, the care necessitated by his condition, he would have made it. Although the course of pathological processes may not have changed, if his life were not otherwise impeded, in all likelihood, he could have extended his life much longer, with some precautions that would have been easy to take.

But the old soldier's dream collapses. Just when he touches the promised land, bereavement and cruelty strike almost at the same time: mobilization occurred and he was recalled to Paris.

We know the role he played and, therefore, his innumerable hardships, his sleepless nights, the obligations of his office, often in opposition to the precautions which had become indispensable for his health. He nevertheless agreed to care for himself, without sacrificing a thing to the terrible duties of his position.

As Minister he now was committed to one of the toughest battles of the campaign when the attention of government and the Ministry of War needed to be more vigilant than ever.

He worked continuously, and, accepting all medical prescriptions which would allow him to function in his office, just tried to "hold on". He pushed himself through his fatigue "without hesitation or murmuring", the endless sessions, the useful and useless, of the House, the long meetings of the Council of Ministers, those of the Commission of the Army, and entertaining endless members of Parliament. It is certainly understandable that, when finally alone with a few friends, he admits to a few complaints, and involuntary cries from a body that truly suffers, but which are quickly suppressed by the energy of a soul which was always master of the body it animated. But fatigue is a slow and insidious poison, accumulating and depleting his force; the General tried new treatments in the hope that he would eventually endure, without having to submit to the pain and leave his post. Not that he was driven by any glory - those who knew him well knew what he thought of Fame. One day, alluding to suspicions that some had conceived about him: "Ambition!" he cried, "Me, ambitious!? They do not know me."

Then, changing his mind: "By the way," he said, "if I am ambitious, I am ambitious for my country! She is all my ambition."

Finally, exhausted and resolved that he will fall and rise no more, he left the Department.

Others had, in his place, previously resorted to rest, and they were so right! But he was a soldier and he will not cease to be: the battle rages, he wished to go back as soon as possible. And then he asked "his doctors" - as he said - if an operation would be able to get him back on his feet. He did not ignore the risks, but it matters little as long as he had a promising chance to get healed and ready to serve his fatherland. His iron will and strength so many times proved his character, the clarity and integrity of his brain so wonderfully organized, were they not reliable guarantors of the future? His doctors thought like him. The intervention will be attempted.

Or, despite the most legitimate expectations, despite the optimum medical conditions for the operation, his body did not take long to be wore down, so unanticipated, the spirit that animated him tried with all its might to revitalize himself, but in vain...

General Gallieni passed away as he had wished, for his country, in full sacrifice, right up to the end, as only a soldier can give.

www.ingramcontent.com/pod-product-compliance
Lightning Source LLC
Chambersburg PA
CBHW052333220526
45472CB00001B/403